NATURAL AND PERMANENT CURE TO LOW SPERM COUNT

Natural And Holistic Methods To Help Men Improve Their Sperm Count, Quality, And Fertility

Dr. Fredrick Kim

TABLE OF CONTNETS

INTRODUCTION

Low sperm count, or oligospermia, is a condition that affects many men worldwide, impacting their fertility and ability to conceive. While it's common to focus on infertility as a women's issue, male fertility plays an equally significant role in conception. Understanding and addressing low sperm count naturally is not only possible but can lead to long-term improvements in sperm health and overall reproductive function.

In this book, we delve into natural and holistic methods to help men improve their sperm count and quality. Whether you're seeking to enhance fertility, support your reproductive health, or prevent the potential risks of low sperm count, this guide offers practical, science-backed approaches that focus on lifestyle, nutrition, exercise, and alternative remedies.

Understanding Low Sperm Count
Sperm count is defined as the concentration of sperm in a man's ejaculate. A normal sperm count is typically above 15 million sperm per milliliter of semen. When sperm count falls below this threshold, it can cause challenges with conception. However, a low sperm count does not mean infertility is inevitable. Many men with low sperm

count can still father children with the right interventions.

There are numerous causes of low sperm count, which may include hormonal imbalances, genetic factors, infections, varicocele (enlarged veins in the scrotum), environmental factors (such as exposure to toxins), and unhealthy lifestyle choices. In some cases, low sperm count may be a result of a combination of these factors.

Causes and Risk Factors for Low Sperm Count
Low sperm count can stem from a variety of causes, and understanding these factors is essential for effective treatment. Some common risk factors include:

Lifestyle Choices: Smoking, excessive alcohol consumption, and poor dietary habits can all lead to a decline in sperm quality.
Environmental Toxins: Exposure to chemicals, heavy metals, and endocrine-disrupting substances can damage sperm production.
Age: Sperm quality can decrease as men age, particularly after the age of 40.
Medical Conditions: Diabetes, obesity, and hormonal imbalances (such as low testosterone) can negatively affect sperm production.
Infections: Certain infections, such as sexually transmitted infections (STIs), can damage the reproductive organs and lower sperm count.

The Importance of Natural Remedies
Conventional treatments for low sperm count often involve medications, surgery, or assisted reproductive technologies (ART) like in-vitro fertilization (IVF). However, many men prefer to explore natural methods first, aiming to improve their fertility without relying on invasive procedures.

Natural remedies offer a holistic approach, focusing on lifestyle improvements, nutrition, and supplementation to enhance overall reproductive health. These methods are not only effective but also support long-term health and wellness, making them an ideal choice for those looking for sustainable solutions.

In the chapters ahead, we will explore a variety of natural and proven ways to increase sperm count. These strategies will help you improve your reproductive health naturally, with minimal side effects. From dietary changes to stress management and herbal remedies, this guide is designed to empower you with the knowledge and tools to take control of your fertility and health.

CHAPTER 1
Nutrition for Sperm Health

A well-balanced, nutrient-rich diet is one of the most effective ways to improve sperm health and count. The foods we eat play a crucial role in the production of sperm and the overall health of the reproductive system. Certain nutrients are essential for promoting healthy sperm production, enhancing motility, and improving sperm quality. By incorporating specific foods and nutrients into your diet, you can support your fertility naturally.

The Role of a Balanced Diet

A healthy, balanced diet ensures that your body receives all the essential vitamins, minerals, and macronutrients needed to produce healthy sperm. Poor nutrition, on the other hand, can lead to deficiencies that negatively impact sperm production. A diet rich in antioxidants, healthy fats, vitamins, and minerals can reduce oxidative stress, balance hormones, and improve sperm motility.

Key Nutrients for Sperm Production

Zinc:

Zinc is one of the most important minerals for male fertility. It is crucial for testosterone production and the formation of sperm cells. Zinc deficiency is linked

to low sperm count, poor sperm motility, and abnormal sperm shape.
Sources: Oysters, beef, pumpkin seeds, lentils, chickpeas, and spinach.

Vitamin C:
As a powerful antioxidant, vitamin C protects sperm from oxidative damage and improves sperm motility. It can also help increase sperm count by improving the overall health of sperm cells.
Sources: Oranges, strawberries, bell peppers, broccoli, and kiwi.

Vitamin E:
Vitamin E is another antioxidant that helps protect sperm from oxidative damage. It also supports sperm cell membrane integrity, which is vital for proper motility and fertilization ability.
Sources: Almonds, sunflower seeds, spinach, avocados, and olive oil.

Folic Acid (Vitamin B9):
Folic acid is essential for DNA synthesis and the formation of healthy sperm. It has been shown to improve sperm count and motility. Men with low folic acid levels are more likely to have sperm with chromosomal abnormalities.
Sources: Leafy greens (spinach, kale), beans, asparagus, and fortified cereals.

Selenium:

Selenium is another antioxidant that plays a role in protecting sperm from oxidative stress. It also helps improve sperm motility and quality.
Sources: Brazil nuts, sunflower seeds, fish (salmon, tuna), and whole grains.

L-Carnitine:
L-carnitine is an amino acid that helps with sperm motility and energy. It is essential for the proper functioning of sperm cells and has been shown to increase sperm count in some men.
Sources: Red meat, poultry, fish, and dairy products.

Omega-3 Fatty Acids:
Omega-3 fatty acids are crucial for hormone regulation and the production of healthy sperm. They help reduce inflammation in the body and improve sperm motility.
Sources: Fatty fish (salmon, mackerel), flaxseeds, chia seeds, and walnuts.

Coenzyme Q10 (CoQ10):
CoQ10 is an antioxidant that supports energy production in sperm cells and helps improve sperm count and motility. It is especially important for older men looking to enhance fertility.
Sources: Meat, fish, spinach, broccoli, and whole grains.

Foods to Boost Sperm Count and Quality
Leafy Greens and Vegetables:

Vegetables such as spinach, kale, and broccoli are rich in folate, vitamins, and antioxidants that protect sperm and enhance fertility.

Berries:
Berries like strawberries, blueberries, and raspberries are packed with antioxidants, particularly vitamin C, which helps improve sperm motility.

Nuts and Seeds:
Almonds, walnuts, sunflower seeds, and pumpkin seeds are excellent sources of healthy fats, zinc, and vitamin E, which promote healthy sperm production.

Whole Grains:
Whole grains such as quinoa, brown rice, and oats are rich in fiber, selenium, and B vitamins, which are essential for hormone balance and sperm health.

Citrus Fruits:
Citrus fruits like oranges, grapefruits, and lemons are rich in vitamin C, which helps protect sperm from oxidative stress and supports sperm motility.

Fatty Fish:
Fatty fish like salmon, mackerel, and sardines are rich in omega-3 fatty acids, which promote healthy sperm motility and reduce inflammation.

Eggs:

Eggs are a great source of protein and vitamin E, both of which are vital for sperm production and quality.

Oysters:
Oysters are one of the richest sources of zinc, which is essential for sperm production and testosterone levels.

Supplements for Male Fertility
In addition to a healthy diet, certain supplements can help fill in any nutritional gaps and improve sperm health:
Zinc Supplements: Zinc plays a crucial role in sperm production, and supplementation may help increase sperm count in men with a deficiency.
Folic Acid: Supplementing with folic acid can help improve sperm count and motility.
Omega-3 Supplements: If you're not getting enough omega-3 fatty acids from your diet, consider taking a fish oil or flaxseed oil supplement.
CoQ10: Supplementing with CoQ10 may help boost sperm count and motility, especially in older men.

Foods and Nutrients to Avoid
Just as certain foods and nutrients can improve sperm health, others can negatively affect sperm production. To optimize sperm count, it's important to avoid:

Trans Fats: Found in processed foods, fried foods, and baked goods, trans fats can reduce sperm quality.
Excessive Alcohol: Heavy drinking can decrease sperm count and motility.
Soy Products: High consumption of soy may disrupt hormone levels due to its estrogen-like compounds.
Caffeine: While moderate caffeine intake is generally safe, excessive caffeine consumption can negatively affect sperm quality.

By incorporating these foods and nutrients into your diet, you can significantly improve your sperm health, motility, and overall fertility. The key is consistency—making these dietary changes part of your everyday lifestyle will help support your reproductive health in the long term.

CHAPTER 2
Herbal and Natural Remedies

Herbal remedies have been used for centuries to support male fertility and improve reproductive health. Many herbs contain compounds that can enhance sperm production, boost sperm motility, and improve overall fertility. These natural remedies work by balancing hormones, reducing oxidative stress, improving circulation, and promoting the health of reproductive organs.

Introduction to Herbal Medicine

Herbal medicine involves the use of plants or plant extracts to treat health conditions. For male fertility, several herbs have been identified for their positive effects on sperm count and quality. These herbs are typically available in the form of capsules, powders, teas, or tinctures, and can be used alone or in combination with other treatments.

Effective Herbal Remedies for Low Sperm Count

Ashwagandha (Withania somnifera)

Benefits: Ashwagandha, also known as Indian ginseng, is one of the most widely used herbs in Ayurvedic medicine. It is known for its stress-reducing properties, which can help lower cortisol levels—a hormone that can negatively affect sperm production. Ashwagandha has also been shown to increase sperm count, motility, and testosterone levels.

How it Works: Ashwagandha helps regulate the endocrine system, promoting hormone balance and improving the health of sperm cells.

Dosage: 300–500 mg of ashwagandha extract per day, taken with water or milk.

Tribulus Terrestris

Benefits: Tribulus Terrestris is a popular herb used to enhance male fertility. It is believed to increase testosterone levels, improve sperm count, and enhance sperm motility.

How it Works: Tribulus works by stimulating the release of luteinizing hormone (LH), which in turn stimulates the production of testosterone. This hormonal boost can result in improved sperm production.

Dosage: 250–500 mg per day, typically taken with meals.

Maca Root (Lepidium meyenii)

Benefits: Maca root is a powerful adaptogen that has been traditionally used to enhance male fertility, increase libido, and improve sperm quality. Studies have shown that maca can increase sperm count and motility, making it a valuable supplement for improving fertility.

How it Works: Maca root works by nourishing the endocrine system, balancing hormone levels, and improving overall energy and vitality. It is also

believed to have a positive effect on sperm production by increasing blood flow to the reproductive organs.
Dosage: 1–3 grams of powdered maca root per day.

Fenugreek (Trigonella foenum-graecum)
Benefits: Fenugreek is another herb that is often used to improve male fertility. It has been shown to increase sperm count and motility, as well as enhance testosterone production.
How it Works: Fenugreek contains compounds called saponins, which have been shown to improve testosterone levels and enhance sexual function. It may also improve the overall health of sperm cells.
Dosage: 500 mg of fenugreek extract per day, often combined with other fertility supplements.

Ginseng (Panax ginseng)
Benefits: Ginseng is one of the most well-known herbs for boosting energy and vitality. It has also been found to improve sperm quality, increase sperm count, and enhance sperm motility.
How it Works: Ginseng works by improving blood flow to the reproductive organs, increasing testosterone levels, and reducing oxidative stress. It also helps improve overall energy and stamina.
Dosage: 200–400 mg of ginseng extract per day.

Saw Palmetto (Serenoa repens)
Benefits: Saw palmetto is known for its ability to support prostate health, but it also has a positive

impact on male fertility. It is often used to enhance sperm count and improve sperm motility.

How it Works: Saw palmetto works by supporting the hormonal system, particularly by balancing the levels of testosterone and dihydrotestosterone (DHT), which can impact sperm production.

Dosage: 320 mg of saw palmetto extract per day.

Shatavari (Asparagus racemosus)

Benefits: Shatavari is another important herb in Ayurvedic medicine that is known for its fertility-enhancing properties. It has been traditionally used to improve reproductive health and increase sperm count.

How it Works: Shatavari works by nourishing the reproductive system, improving hormonal balance, and supporting the production of healthy sperm.

Dosage: 500 mg to 1 gram of shatavari powder per day.

Tongkat Ali (Eurycoma longifolia)

Benefits: Tongkat Ali, also known as Malaysian ginseng, is a popular herb used to improve testosterone levels, enhance libido, and boost sperm quality.

How it Works: Tongkat Ali works by stimulating the production of luteinizing hormone (LH), which increases testosterone production. It has also been shown to improve sperm motility and overall fertility.

Dosage: 200–300 mg of Tongkat Ali extract per day.

Pygeum (Prunus africana)
Benefits: Pygeum is commonly used to support prostate health, but it also has a positive effect on male fertility. It has been shown to increase sperm count and improve the overall health of sperm.
How it Works: Pygeum helps regulate hormonal balance and improve prostate function, which can positively influence sperm production.
Dosage: 100–200 mg of pygeum extract per day.

Other Natural Remedies
In addition to herbal treatments, other natural remedies may help improve sperm count and quality:

L-Carnitine: An amino acid that helps improve sperm motility. It can be found in foods like red meat and fish, or taken as a supplement.

Coenzyme Q10 (CoQ10): A powerful antioxidant that supports energy production in sperm cells and enhances sperm motility and count.

Acupuncture: Some studies suggest that acupuncture can help improve sperm count and quality by improving circulation and balancing hormones.

Moringa (Moringa oleifera): A nutrient-dense plant that has been used for its potential to improve sperm count and motility. It is also rich in vitamins and antioxidants.

Herbal and natural remedies offer a holistic and effective approach to improving sperm count and quality. Many of these herbs have been used for centuries in traditional medicine, and modern research continues to support their use for enhancing male fertility. However, it's important to consult with a healthcare professional before starting any herbal supplements to ensure safety and effectiveness. Combining these natural remedies with a healthy diet, regular exercise, and stress management can provide a comprehensive approach to improving fertility and achieving better reproductive health.

CHAPTER 3
Lifestyle Modifications

A healthy lifestyle plays a crucial role in maintaining optimal sperm count and overall fertility. Making intentional changes to daily habits can significantly improve sperm health. From regular physical activity to stress management and sleep, various lifestyle modifications have been proven to positively affect sperm quality and production.

The Impact of Lifestyle on Sperm Health

Several lifestyle factors can either positively or negatively impact sperm health. Factors such as diet, exercise, alcohol consumption, smoking, and stress levels all contribute to sperm count, motility, and quality. Making the right lifestyle choices is essential for improving fertility and overall well-being.

Exercise and Physical Activity

Regular exercise is one of the most effective ways to improve sperm health. Physical activity helps to balance hormone levels, improve blood flow to the reproductive organs, and reduce stress. However, it's essential to strike a balance—while moderate exercise is beneficial, excessive exercise or overtraining can lead to a decline in sperm quality.

Benefits of Exercise:
Increases testosterone levels
Improves circulation, ensuring better blood flow to the testicles
Helps reduce oxidative stress, which can damage sperm
Supports weight management, which can prevent obesity-related fertility issues

Recommended Activities:
Moderate Aerobic Exercise: Activities such as jogging, swimming, cycling, or walking for 30 minutes a day can boost sperm count and overall health.
Strength Training: Weight lifting or resistance training a few times a week can help maintain muscle mass and support hormonal balance.
Yoga: Yoga is beneficial for both physical and mental health. Certain poses (like those that promote relaxation and circulation) may support reproductive health.

Exercise to Avoid:
Overtraining: Excessive endurance exercise (like marathon running or high-intensity sports) can lead to increased cortisol levels, which can negatively affect sperm production.
Overheating: Avoid exercises or activities that cause excessive sweating and overheating of the testicles, as this can damage sperm production.

Weight Management
Maintaining a healthy weight is one of the most important factors for improving sperm health. Both overweight and underweight men may experience reduced fertility due to hormonal imbalances, poor sperm production, or reduced motility.

Obesity and Male Fertility: Excess weight, especially around the abdomen, can disrupt hormone levels, leading to lower testosterone production. Obesity is also linked to oxidative stress and inflammation, which can damage sperm cells.

Underweight and Fertility: Being underweight can also negatively affect sperm production by causing low energy levels and hormonal imbalances, leading to reduced fertility.

Weight Loss Tips:
Focus on a balanced diet rich in whole foods, including vegetables, fruits, lean proteins, and healthy fats.
Incorporate regular exercise to maintain a healthy weight and reduce fat buildup around the abdomen.

Stress Reduction
Chronic stress can have a significant impact on sperm production. High levels of cortisol (the stress hormone) can disrupt testosterone production, leading to decreased sperm count and motility. Additionally, stress can interfere with healthy sleep

patterns and contribute to unhealthy lifestyle choices, which can further impact fertility.

How Stress Affects Fertility:
Chronic stress leads to hormonal imbalances, which can impair sperm production and quality.
Elevated cortisol levels reduce testosterone, negatively impacting both sperm count and motility.

Stress Management Techniques:
Meditation: Mindfulness and relaxation meditation can reduce stress and promote emotional well-being, improving overall fertility.
Deep Breathing Exercises: Breathing exercises, such as diaphragmatic breathing or the 4-7-8 technique, help reduce tension and promote relaxation.
Journaling or Talking to Someone: Expressing emotions and talking through stressful situations can help reduce mental and emotional strain.
Time in Nature: Spending time outdoors, whether through a walk in the park or a nature hike, has been shown to reduce stress and improve mood.

Sleep Quality
Quality sleep is vital for maintaining healthy testosterone levels and overall fertility. Studies have shown that men who do not get enough sleep (less than 7 hours per night) have lower sperm count, motility, and poor sperm quality.

Benefits of Good Sleep:
Testosterone production peaks during deep sleep. A lack of quality rest can lead to lower testosterone levels and reduced sperm production.
Proper sleep helps regulate the body's hormone levels, promoting better sperm health.

Sleep Tips:
Aim for 7-8 hours of sleep each night, ideally between 10:00 PM and 6:00 AM.
Create a Sleep Routine: Going to bed and waking up at the same time every day helps regulate your body's internal clock.
Limit Blue Light Exposure: Avoid screens (phones, tablets, computers, TVs) at least an hour before bed to improve the quality of sleep.
Sleep Environment: Keep your bedroom cool, dark, and quiet to create a relaxing sleep environment.

Avoiding Harmful Substances
Certain substances can negatively impact sperm count and overall fertility. Avoiding or reducing exposure to harmful chemicals, drugs, and lifestyle choices can significantly enhance sperm health.

Alcohol Consumption: Excessive alcohol intake can lead to reduced sperm count, lower testosterone levels, and poor sperm motility. Limiting alcohol consumption is essential for improving fertility.

Recommendation: Limit alcohol to no more than 1–2 drinks per week.

Smoking: Smoking has been shown to decrease sperm count, motility, and overall sperm quality. It also increases the risk of DNA fragmentation in sperm, leading to possible fertility issues.

Recommendation: Quit smoking to significantly improve sperm quality and reproductive health.

Environmental Toxins: Exposure to environmental toxins such as pesticides, plastics, heavy metals (lead, mercury), and endocrine-disrupting chemicals can interfere with sperm production and overall fertility.

Recommendation: Reduce exposure by opting for organic foods when possible, avoiding plastic containers for food storage, and using natural cleaning products.

Recreational Drugs: The use of recreational drugs, such as marijuana and cocaine, can negatively affect sperm count and motility.

Recommendation: Avoid the use of recreational drugs to protect your fertility.

Testicular Health

Maintaining healthy testicles is crucial for sperm production. Several lifestyle changes can help maintain optimal testicular health and ensure proper sperm production.

Avoid Overheating: The testicles function best at a temperature slightly lower than the body's core temperature. Avoid activities that can overheat the testicles, such as sitting in hot tubs or using laptops on your lap for extended periods.
Wear Loose-Fitting Underwear: Tight underwear and pants can increase the temperature around the testicles, reducing sperm production. Opt for loose-fitting boxers over tight briefs to maintain healthy sperm production.

Relationship Health
A positive and supportive relationship can reduce stress, improve emotional well-being, and support overall health, including fertility. Open communication with your partner about family planning, emotional support, and lifestyle choices can help you work together to achieve optimal fertility.

Lifestyle modifications are an essential part of improving sperm health and fertility. By adopting healthy habits, managing stress, maintaining a balanced weight, and avoiding harmful substances, you can naturally enhance your sperm count and quality. Incorporating these lifestyle changes along with dietary and herbal interventions will provide a comprehensive approach to improving your reproductive health, increasing your chances of conception, and maintaining overall well-being.

CHAPTER 4

Environmental Factors and Toxins

Environmental factors and toxins can have a significant impact on male fertility. Many modern lifestyle habits expose individuals to harmful chemicals, pollutants, and endocrine-disrupting substances that can negatively affect sperm health. These environmental toxins can disrupt hormone levels, reduce sperm count, impair sperm motility, and even cause DNA damage in sperm. Understanding and minimizing exposure to these harmful factors is crucial for improving sperm health and fertility.

The Impact of Environmental Toxins on Sperm Health

Environmental toxins can interfere with the body's normal functioning and negatively impact sperm production in several ways:

Hormonal Disruption: Many environmental toxins act as endocrine disruptors, meaning they can interfere with the production, secretion, and regulation of hormones such as testosterone, estrogen, and thyroid hormones.

Oxidative Stress: Pollutants and toxins can increase oxidative stress in the body, leading to cell damage, including damage to sperm cells.

DNA Fragmentation: Certain chemicals can cause DNA fragmentation in sperm, leading to reduced fertility and an increased risk of miscarriage or birth defects.
Reduced Sperm Count and Quality: Prolonged exposure to toxins can lead to lower sperm counts, decreased sperm motility, and poorer overall sperm quality.

Common Environmental Factors and Toxins Affecting Sperm Count

Endocrine-Disrupting Chemicals (EDCs)
Endocrine-disrupting chemicals (EDCs) are chemicals that interfere with the body's hormonal system. They can mimic, block, or alter the body's natural hormones, leading to imbalances that may affect sperm production.

Common EDCs:
Bisphenol A (BPA): A plasticizer found in many plastics, such as water bottles, food containers, and thermal paper receipts. BPA can mimic estrogen and disrupt hormone levels, leading to reduced sperm quality.
Phthalates: Found in a variety of personal care products (like shampoos, deodorants, and lotions), phthalates are used to make plastics more flexible. They are also linked to reduced sperm count and motility.
Parabens: These chemicals are commonly used as preservatives in cosmetics, lotions, and personal

care products. Parabens have been shown to act like estrogen and may reduce sperm count.
Pesticides and Herbicides: Chemicals used in farming to control pests and weeds can enter the food chain and disrupt endocrine function, leading to decreased sperm health.
How They Affect Fertility: These chemicals can lead to lower testosterone levels, impaired sperm development, and oxidative damage to sperm cells.

Heavy Metals
Heavy metals such as lead, mercury, and cadmium can have harmful effects on reproductive health. These metals are often found in polluted air, water, soil, and even in certain foods like fish.

Lead: Exposure to lead, commonly found in old pipes, paint, and contaminated water, has been linked to reduced sperm count and motility, as well as abnormal sperm morphology (shape).

Mercury: Mercury is found in some fish, especially large predatory fish like tuna and swordfish, and can interfere with sperm production and quality.

Cadmium: Exposure to cadmium, which can come from polluted air, cigarettes, and contaminated food, has been shown to reduce sperm count and motility.

How They Affect Fertility: These metals can cause oxidative stress, hormone disruption, and DNA damage in sperm cells, leading to reduced fertility.

Radiation
Exposure to high levels of radiation can negatively impact sperm production. Sperm cells are particularly sensitive to radiation, and even low doses of radiation can reduce sperm count, motility, and cause DNA fragmentation.

Sources of Radiation:
Cell Phones: The electromagnetic radiation emitted by mobile phones can potentially affect sperm quality. Holding a cell phone in close proximity to the testicles may result in sperm damage.
X-Rays and Medical Imaging: Repeated exposure to radiation from medical imaging (X-rays, CT scans) can negatively affect sperm production.
Environmental Radiation: Living in areas with high levels of environmental radiation, such as near nuclear power plants or contaminated sites, may increase the risk of sperm damage.
How It Affects Fertility: Radiation exposure can lead to DNA damage in sperm, which may reduce fertility and increase the risk of birth defects or miscarriages.

Pollutants in Air and Water
Air and water pollution are significant environmental factors that can harm male fertility. Exposure to air

pollution, including particulate matter (PM), nitrogen dioxide (NO2), and carbon monoxide (CO), can damage sperm quality and reduce sperm count.

Air Pollution: Pollutants in the air can create free radicals and increase oxidative stress, which damages sperm cells.

Water Pollution: Contaminants in drinking water, such as industrial chemicals and heavy metals, can disrupt the endocrine system and affect sperm production.

How It Affects Fertility: Pollutants contribute to oxidative stress, disrupt hormonal balance, and reduce sperm quality.

Workplace Toxins
Certain professions expose workers to harmful chemicals and toxins that can negatively affect sperm health. Jobs that involve exposure to heavy metals, solvents, pesticides, or other harmful chemicals may increase the risk of fertility issues.

Common Occupations at Risk:
Farmers: Exposure to pesticides and herbicides.
Mechanics: Exposure to solvents, oils, and heavy metals.
Construction Workers: Exposure to lead, asbestos, and other industrial chemicals.

Painters and Chemical Workers: Exposure to volatile organic compounds (VOCs) and solvents.
How It Affects Fertility: Workplace toxins can cause oxidative stress, disrupt hormone production, and reduce sperm count and motility.

How to Reduce Exposure to Environmental Toxins

While it may not be possible to completely eliminate exposure to environmental toxins, there are several strategies to reduce contact with harmful substances:

Avoid Plastics and BPA-Containing Products
Use BPA-Free Products: Opt for BPA-free plastics or choose glass, stainless steel, or ceramic containers for food storage.
Avoid Canned Foods: Many canned foods are lined with BPA-containing coatings. Choose fresh or frozen foods instead.
Reduce Use of Thermal Paper: Avoid handling receipts and other items made from thermal paper, which often contain BPA.

Choose Organic Foods
Reduce Pesticide Exposure: Choose organic produce whenever possible to minimize exposure to pesticides and herbicides that can disrupt hormonal balance.

Limit Exposure to Heavy Metals

Choose Fish Wisely: Avoid consuming high-mercury fish like swordfish, shark, and large tuna. Opt for lower-mercury options such as salmon, sardines, and trout.

Check Water Quality: Use a water filter that removes heavy metals and other toxins from drinking water.

Avoid Lead Paint: Ensure that homes and buildings (especially older ones) do not have lead-based paints.

Reduce Radiation Exposure

Limit Cell Phone Use: Avoid carrying your phone in your pocket or near your reproductive organs. Use hands-free options or speakerphone to reduce direct exposure.

Minimize X-Ray Exposure: Limit medical imaging procedures to those that are absolutely necessary. Use alternative methods of diagnosis where possible.

Detoxify Your Living Space

Ventilate Your Home: Ensure your home is well-ventilated to reduce indoor air pollution. Use air purifiers and avoid using chemicals like harsh cleaners or air fresheners that may release toxins into the air.

Choose Natural Products: Opt for natural cleaning products, paints, and personal care items that do not contain harmful chemicals.

Protect Yourself at Work

Use Protective Gear: Wear appropriate protective clothing and equipment when handling chemicals, solvents, or other toxins at work.
Practice Proper Hygiene: Wash hands regularly and shower after exposure to potential toxins, especially when handling pesticides or chemicals.

Environmental toxins and pollutants play a significant role in reducing sperm count, motility, and quality. By understanding the impact of these toxins and making deliberate efforts to reduce exposure, you can take proactive steps to protect your fertility. Reducing contact with endocrine disruptors, heavy metals, pollutants, and radiation can significantly improve sperm health and overall reproductive wellness. Incorporating these practices into your daily life, alongside a healthy lifestyle and proper nutrition, will help you maintain optimal fertility and reproductive health.

CHAPTER 5

The Role of Stress in Sperm Count

Stress is a significant factor that can affect various aspects of health, including male fertility. Chronic stress can negatively impact sperm count, quality, and motility. Stress hormones, particularly cortisol, can disrupt the delicate balance of reproductive hormones, leading to a decrease in sperm production and quality.

How Stress Affects Sperm Health

Stress, particularly chronic or long-term stress, can have several negative effects on male fertility. The primary mechanism through which stress affects sperm count is through the release of the stress hormone cortisol.

Cortisol and Hormonal Imbalance

Cortisol, often called the "stress hormone," is released by the adrenal glands in response to stress. When stress is experienced, the body goes into a "fight-or-flight" mode, preparing to respond to perceived threats. While short-term stress can be beneficial in certain situations, prolonged stress leads to a sustained increase in cortisol levels, which can disrupt the body's hormonal balance, including the production of reproductive hormones such as testosterone.

How It Affects Sperm Production: High cortisol levels inhibit the production of luteinizing hormone (LH) and follicle-stimulating hormone (FSH), both of which are necessary for the stimulation of sperm production in the testes. Chronic stress can reduce the secretion of testosterone, which is critical for the development and maturation of sperm.

Increased Estrogen: Elevated cortisol levels can also lead to an increase in estrogen, a hormone typically associated with female reproduction. High estrogen levels in men can lead to a decrease in sperm count and quality.

Reduced Testosterone: Since cortisol and testosterone share a similar production pathway, prolonged stress can reduce the amount of testosterone available for sperm production, further impairing fertility.

Impaired Sperm Quality
In addition to reducing sperm count, stress can negatively affect sperm quality in several ways:

DNA Fragmentation: Chronic stress has been shown to cause oxidative stress, which occurs when the body produces excessive free radicals. These free radicals can damage sperm DNA, leading to DNA fragmentation. Damaged sperm DNA can reduce fertilization rates and increase the risk of miscarriage and birth defects.

Reduced Sperm Motility: Stress can also impair sperm motility (the ability of sperm to swim and reach the egg). Sperm with poor motility have a lower chance of successfully fertilizing an egg, reducing the likelihood of conception.

Abnormal Sperm Morphology: Stress may contribute to morphological abnormalities in sperm, such as irregular shape or size, which can affect their ability to penetrate and fertilize an egg.

Impact on Semen Volume

Stress has been linked to a reduction in semen volume. Men with chronic stress may produce less semen, which can reduce the number of sperm released during ejaculation. Lower semen volume can be associated with fertility challenges, as the number of sperm in each ejaculation is a key factor in conception.

Reduced Libido and Sexual Function

Chronic stress can lead to sexual dysfunction, including reduced libido and erectile dysfunction (ED). This can further reduce the frequency of sexual activity and the chances of conception. Stress can interfere with the ability to achieve and maintain an erection, while also reducing interest in sex, which compounds fertility issues.

The Effects of Acute vs. Chronic Stress

Not all stress is created equal. Acute stress, such as a temporary stressful event, may have minimal impact on sperm count or quality. However, chronic stress, which persists over a long period, can have a more pronounced and lasting effect on reproductive health.

Acute Stress: Short-term stress, like preparing for a big presentation or dealing with a sudden life event, may cause a temporary increase in cortisol levels. However, this increase typically does not last long enough to have a significant impact on sperm health.
Chronic Stress: Long-term stress, such as ongoing financial worries, relationship issues, or work-related stress, results in consistently elevated cortisol levels. This sustained stress can lead to hormonal imbalances, reduced testosterone production, and long-term fertility issues.

Factors That Exacerbate Stress and Impact Sperm Health
Several factors can exacerbate the negative impact of stress on sperm count and quality:
Poor Sleep
Stress often leads to disrupted sleep patterns, which can further elevate cortisol levels. Lack of sleep and poor-quality sleep are both associated with reduced testosterone production, which can negatively affect sperm count and quality.

Sleep and Stress Connection: Sleep deprivation increases cortisol levels and decreases the production of important fertility hormones, making it more challenging to maintain optimal sperm health.

Poor Diet and Nutrition
Stress can lead to poor dietary choices, such as overeating, consuming unhealthy comfort foods, or drinking excessive caffeine or alcohol. Poor nutrition and unhealthy eating habits can increase oxidative stress, disrupt hormone balance, and reduce sperm quality.

Impact on Fertility: A diet rich in processed foods, unhealthy fats, and sugar can increase inflammation in the body and negatively affect sperm production and quality.

Alcohol and Tobacco Use
Stress often leads to unhealthy coping mechanisms, such as smoking or drinking alcohol. Both smoking and excessive alcohol consumption can negatively affect sperm count, motility, and overall sperm health. These substances are also associated with increased oxidative stress, which can damage sperm.

Smoking: Smoking has been shown to reduce sperm motility and DNA integrity, as well as lower sperm count.
Alcohol: Chronic alcohol consumption is linked to lower testosterone levels, impaired sperm production, and reduced semen quality.

Managing Stress to Improve Sperm Health

Since stress can significantly impact sperm count and fertility, managing and reducing stress is a vital step in improving reproductive health. Below are some effective strategies to manage stress and improve sperm health:

Mindfulness and Meditation
Mindfulness techniques, such as meditation, deep breathing, and progressive muscle relaxation, can help reduce the body's stress response. These practices have been shown to lower cortisol levels and promote emotional well-being.

Mindfulness: Practicing mindfulness encourages relaxation and a sense of calm, which can significantly reduce overall stress levels.
Meditation: Regular meditation, even for a few minutes each day, has been shown to decrease cortisol levels, improve mental clarity, and support reproductive health.

Regular Exercise
Physical activity is one of the most effective ways to reduce stress and improve overall well-being. Exercise helps reduce cortisol levels and stimulates the production of endorphins, the body's natural mood elevators.

Recommended Activities: Moderate aerobic exercises, such as jogging, swimming, or cycling, as well as strength training and yoga, are excellent ways to reduce stress and boost fertility.

Avoid Overtraining: While regular exercise is beneficial, excessive exercise can actually increase stress and harm fertility. It's essential to find a balance.

Quality Sleep

Adequate and quality sleep is essential for reducing stress and improving fertility. A consistent sleep routine helps regulate cortisol levels and allows the body to repair and restore hormone production.

Sleep Hygiene Tips:

Go to bed at the same time each night.

Avoid electronic devices before bedtime to promote better sleep.

Create a relaxing bedtime routine.

Nutritional Support

A healthy diet can help the body cope with stress and support fertility. Nutrient-rich foods can help balance hormones, reduce inflammation, and boost overall reproductive health.

Foods for Stress Relief: Include foods high in omega-3 fatty acids (such as fatty fish), antioxidants (fruits and vegetables), and vitamins and minerals

(magnesium, zinc) that help reduce inflammation and support hormone balance.
Avoid Caffeine and Sugar: Excessive caffeine and sugar intake can exacerbate stress and disrupt hormone production. Limit these to help manage stress more effectively.

Professional Support and Therapy
If stress is overwhelming, seeking professional support from a therapist or counselor can be incredibly beneficial. Cognitive-behavioral therapy (CBT), for example, can help individuals manage stress, anxiety, and other mental health issues that may affect fertility.

Social Support
Maintaining strong relationships with friends, family, and partners is crucial for emotional support. Having a support system can help buffer against stress and provide comfort during difficult times.

Stress plays a significant role in male fertility, affecting sperm count, quality, and overall reproductive health. Chronic stress increases cortisol levels, which disrupts hormonal balance, reduces testosterone, and impairs sperm production. Managing stress through mindfulness, exercise, sleep, nutrition, and professional support can help reduce cortisol levels and improve sperm health. Taking proactive steps to minimize stress is a key part of improving fertility and enhancing overall well-being.

CHAPTER 6

The Power of Sleep and Hydration

Sleep and hydration are two fundamental aspects of overall health that directly influence sperm count, quality, and fertility. Adequate sleep and proper hydration play essential roles in maintaining hormonal balance, reducing oxidative stress, and supporting reproductive health.

The Role of Sleep in Sperm Health

Sleep is crucial for both physical and mental well-being. For male fertility, sleep plays an especially important role in regulating hormone production, supporting cellular repair, and reducing stress—all of which directly impact sperm health.

Hormonal Balance and Testosterone Production
Adequate sleep is essential for the production of hormones, particularly testosterone, which plays a critical role in sperm production. Testosterone levels naturally fluctuate throughout the day, peaking in the early morning hours and decreasing throughout the day. Sleep, especially during the deeper stages of the sleep cycle, is when the body produces the highest levels of testosterone.

Testosterone Production: Research has shown that even short-term sleep deprivation can lead to a significant decrease in testosterone levels. Low testosterone levels are linked to reduced sperm count and quality.

Sleep and Follicle-Stimulating Hormone (FSH): FSH, which stimulates sperm production in the testes, is also influenced by sleep patterns. Sleep disruption can interfere with the secretion of FSH, further affecting sperm production.

Sleep and Sperm Quality
Sleep also impacts sperm motility (the ability of sperm to move efficiently) and sperm morphology (the size and shape of sperm). Poor sleep can result in a decline in both of these important sperm characteristics.

Sperm Motility: Men who experience chronic sleep deprivation or poor-quality sleep tend to have sperm with lower motility. This can make it more difficult for sperm to travel through the female reproductive tract and reach the egg.
Sperm Morphology: Sleep deprivation has been linked to an increase in sperm abnormalities. A lack of proper sleep can contribute to irregularities in sperm shape, which may affect the sperm's ability to fertilize an egg.

Sleep and Oxidative Stress
Oxidative stress occurs when the body produces an excess of free radicals, which can damage cells, including sperm cells. Sleep plays a crucial role in

reducing oxidative stress by allowing the body to repair itself and restore balance. Poor sleep, on the other hand, increases oxidative stress, which can negatively impact sperm DNA and motility.

Oxidative Damage: Chronic lack of sleep increases oxidative stress in the body, which can lead to sperm DNA fragmentation—a condition where the DNA inside sperm cells becomes damaged. DNA fragmentation can reduce the chances of successful fertilization and increase the risk of miscarriage.

Sleep and Overall Health
Sleep is essential for maintaining overall health, including the immune system, metabolism, and stress regulation. Poor sleep is linked to a range of health issues such as obesity, diabetes, high blood pressure, and depression—all of which can affect fertility. By getting enough rest, the body is better able to maintain a healthy reproductive system and optimal sperm production.

How Much Sleep Do You Need?
The ideal amount of sleep for fertility and overall health can vary by individual, but most adults require between 7 to 9 hours of sleep per night for optimal functioning. Consistently getting enough rest helps ensure that testosterone levels remain balanced, reduces stress, and allows the body to repair and restore vital systems, including those responsible for reproductive health.

Sleep Quality: It's not just about the number of hours spent sleeping, but also the quality of sleep. Sleep cycles consist of different stages, including deep sleep (REM sleep), which is essential for hormone production and cellular repair. It's important to prioritize uninterrupted, restful sleep for the best fertility outcomes.

Sleep Consistency: Going to bed and waking up at the same time each day helps regulate the body's internal clock, or circadian rhythm. Consistency in sleep patterns is important for hormone regulation and overall health.

The Role of Hydration in Sperm Health

Proper hydration is another essential factor in maintaining optimal sperm health. The human body is composed mostly of water, and staying well-hydrated supports nearly every physiological function, including digestion, circulation, and cellular repair. For reproductive health, hydration plays a crucial role in sperm production, semen quality, and overall fertility.

Hydration and Semen Volume

The fluid portion of semen is largely composed of water, which is essential for maintaining semen volume and supporting sperm motility. Dehydration can lead to a decrease in semen volume, which can reduce the number of sperm in each ejaculation and impair fertility.

Low Semen Volume: Studies have shown that dehydration can lead to lower semen volume, which in turn reduces the total sperm count in each ejaculate. A decrease in semen volume can also make it more difficult for sperm to reach the egg.
Thicker Semen: Inadequate hydration can result in thicker, more viscous semen. This can make it more difficult for sperm to swim and reach the egg, potentially decreasing the chances of conception.

Hydration and Sperm Quality
In addition to influencing semen volume, hydration also affects the quality of sperm. Proper hydration helps maintain the health of sperm cells and supports optimal sperm motility and morphology.

Sperm Motility: Well-hydrated sperm are better able to move efficiently, which is crucial for navigating the female reproductive tract and reaching the egg. Dehydration can impair sperm motility and reduce the chances of successful fertilization.
Sperm Shape and Size: Hydration helps maintain proper cellular function and structure, ensuring that sperm cells remain healthy and maintain an optimal shape for fertilization.

Hydration and Detoxification
Water plays a vital role in the body's ability to detoxify and remove waste products. Proper hydration helps the kidneys flush out toxins and

metabolic waste products that can otherwise accumulate in the body and affect sperm production.

Detoxification: Staying hydrated supports the body's natural detoxification processes, helping to remove harmful substances that can negatively impact sperm health. This includes eliminating excess estrogen or other chemicals that may disrupt the balance of reproductive hormones.

How Much Water Should You Drink?

The ideal amount of water needed for optimal hydration can vary depending on individual factors such as body size, activity level, and climate. However, a general recommendation is to drink at least 8 cups (64 ounces) of water per day. Some individuals may need more water if they are physically active or live in hot climates.

Monitor Urine Color: A simple way to gauge hydration is to observe the color of your urine. Clear or pale yellow urine indicates proper hydration, while dark yellow or amber-colored urine may indicate dehydration.

How to Optimize Sleep and Hydration for Better Sperm Health

Sleep Optimization Tips

Create a Sleep-Friendly Environment: Make your bedroom conducive to sleep by keeping it dark, cool, and quiet. Consider using blackout curtains or an eye mask to block out light.

Limit Stimulants: Avoid caffeine, nicotine, or alcohol before bed, as these can disrupt sleep patterns and affect the quality of your rest.

Practice Relaxation Techniques: Engage in calming activities before bed, such as reading, listening to soothing music, or practicing deep breathing exercises to help relax your body and mind.

Hydration Optimization Tips

Drink Water Consistently: Aim to drink water throughout the day rather than consuming large amounts all at once. Carry a water bottle with you to remind yourself to stay hydrated.

Avoid Excessive Caffeine and Alcohol: Both caffeine and alcohol can have a diuretic effect, leading to increased urination and dehydration. Limit your intake of these beverages to maintain optimal hydration.

Eat Hydrating Foods: In addition to drinking water, include water-rich foods in your diet, such as fruits (e.g., watermelon, cucumbers, oranges) and vegetables (e.g., celery, spinach, tomatoes), to boost hydration.

Sleep and hydration are two powerful factors that contribute to optimal sperm health. Adequate sleep supports hormonal balance, reduces oxidative stress, and enhances sperm quality, while proper hydration is essential for maintaining semen volume, sperm motility, and overall reproductive health. By prioritizing both sleep and hydration, men can improve their fertility and increase their chances of conception. Making small, consistent changes to sleep habits and hydration practices can have a profound impact on reproductive health and overall well-being.

CHAPTER 7

Habits to Avoid

Certain lifestyle habits can have a negative impact on sperm count, quality, and overall fertility. It's important to be mindful of these habits and make changes to improve reproductive health.

Smoking

Smoking is one of the most harmful habits for male fertility. The chemicals in tobacco, such as nicotine and carbon monoxide, can reduce sperm count, impair motility, and increase sperm abnormalities. Smoking also contributes to oxidative stress, which can damage sperm DNA and reduce overall sperm health.

How Smoking Affects Sperm Health:
Reduced Sperm Count: Studies show that smoking is associated with lower sperm count. Smoking affects the production of sperm in the testes, reducing overall sperm quantity.
Impaired Sperm Motility: Smoking damages sperm cells, affecting their ability to swim efficiently toward the egg. Poor motility can significantly lower the chances of successful fertilization.
DNA Damage: Chemicals in tobacco smoke cause oxidative stress, leading to DNA fragmentation in sperm cells. DNA damage is linked to reduced

fertility and higher risks of miscarriage or birth defects.

How to Avoid Smoking:
Seek Support: Consider joining a smoking cessation program or working with a healthcare professional to develop a plan to quit smoking.
Nicotine Replacement: If necessary, use nicotine replacement therapies (e.g., patches or gum) to help manage cravings while quitting.
Supportive Environment: Surround yourself with a supportive environment, including friends, family, or support groups, to help you stay committed to quitting.

Excessive Alcohol Consumption
Excessive alcohol consumption can significantly impact sperm health. While moderate alcohol intake may not have a major effect, heavy drinking can reduce sperm count, impair motility, and increase the risk of erectile dysfunction (ED).

How Alcohol Affects Sperm Health:
Hormonal Disruption: Excessive alcohol consumption can disrupt the balance of reproductive hormones, leading to lower testosterone levels. This can reduce sperm production and quality.
Sperm Motility and Morphology: Alcohol reduces sperm motility and increases the likelihood of sperm abnormalities. This can decrease the chances of successful fertilization.

Testicular Function: Chronic alcohol use can lead to reduced testicular function and damage to sperm-producing cells, leading to lower sperm count.

How to Avoid Excessive Alcohol Consumption:
Limit Intake: If you choose to drink, limit alcohol intake to no more than 1-2 drinks per day. The less alcohol you consume, the less it will impact sperm health.
Choose Healthier Alternatives: If you are struggling with reducing alcohol consumption, try drinking non-alcoholic beverages or replacing alcohol with healthier options like sparkling water or herbal teas.
Seek Professional Help: If alcohol consumption is becoming problematic, consider seeking support from a counselor or a support group to help reduce or eliminate alcohol use.

Excessive Heat Exposure
Prolonged exposure to high temperatures can negatively impact sperm production. The testes are located outside the body for a reason: they need to be kept cooler than the rest of the body for optimal sperm production. Exposure to excessive heat from hot tubs, saunas, tight clothing, or laptops placed directly on the lap can impair sperm count and quality.

How Heat Affects Sperm Health:
Reduced Sperm Production: Heat can affect the temperature of the testes, leading to a decrease in

sperm production. The optimal temperature for sperm production is slightly lower than body temperature.

Decreased Sperm Motility: Heat exposure can reduce sperm motility, making it harder for sperm to swim toward and fertilize an egg.

Damage to Sperm Cells: Long-term heat exposure can damage sperm cells, leading to abnormalities in shape and structure.

How to Avoid Excessive Heat Exposure:

Avoid Hot Environments: Limit the use of hot tubs, saunas, or steam rooms, as the heat can impair sperm health.

Wear Loose Clothing: Avoid tight underwear, jeans, or pants that can increase the temperature around the testes. Opt for loose-fitting, breathable clothing to help keep the area cool.

Laptop Use: Avoid placing a laptop directly on your lap for extended periods, as the heat generated by the device can raise the temperature of the testes.

Poor Diet and Unhealthy Eating Habits

A poor diet can have a detrimental effect on sperm health. Diets that are high in processed foods, unhealthy fats, and sugar can lead to inflammation, hormonal imbalances, and reduced sperm quality. Conversely, a nutrient-dense diet rich in vitamins, minerals, and antioxidants supports healthy sperm production and quality.

How Poor Diet Affects Sperm Health:
Increased Oxidative Stress: Diets high in processed foods and trans fats contribute to oxidative stress, which can damage sperm DNA and reduce sperm motility.
Hormonal Imbalance: Diets that are high in sugar and refined carbohydrates can lead to insulin resistance, which disrupts the balance of hormones necessary for sperm production.
Nutrient Deficiency: A lack of essential vitamins and minerals, such as zinc, folate, and vitamin C, can impair sperm quality and motility.

How to Avoid Poor Diet and Unhealthy Eating Habits:
Choose Whole Foods: Focus on whole, unprocessed foods like fruits, vegetables, lean proteins, and whole grains to provide the nutrients needed for healthy sperm production.
Limit Processed Foods: Avoid or limit the consumption of processed foods, refined sugars, and trans fats, as these can contribute to inflammation and hormonal imbalances.
Eat Antioxidant-Rich Foods: Incorporate foods rich in antioxidants, such as berries, nuts, and leafy greens, to combat oxidative stress and protect sperm from damage.

Lack of Physical Activity
Sedentary behavior and a lack of physical activity can negatively affect sperm health. Regular exercise

is important for maintaining a healthy weight, regulating hormones, and reducing stress—factors that contribute to improved fertility.

How Lack of Exercise Affects Sperm Health:
Obesity and Sperm Health: Being overweight or obese is associated with lower testosterone levels, reduced sperm count, and decreased sperm motility. Excess fat, particularly abdominal fat, increases the production of estrogen, which can further disrupt sperm production.
Reduced Circulation: Physical activity promotes better circulation, which is essential for delivering nutrients and oxygen to the reproductive organs, supporting healthy sperm production.

How to Avoid Sedentary Behavior:
Exercise Regularly: Aim for at least 30 minutes of moderate exercise most days of the week. Activities like walking, jogging, cycling, or swimming can improve circulation, boost testosterone levels, and support overall health.
Strength Training: Incorporate strength training exercises, such as weight lifting, to increase muscle mass and improve hormonal balance.
Avoid Long Periods of Sitting: If you have a sedentary job or lifestyle, make it a habit to stand up, stretch, and move around every hour.

Chronic Stress

Chronic stress can disrupt hormonal balance, reduce testosterone levels, and impair sperm production. The stress hormone cortisol negatively affects sperm count, motility, and overall sperm health. Managing stress is essential for maintaining fertility.

How Stress Affects Sperm Health:
Hormonal Disruption: Chronic stress increases cortisol levels, which can inhibit the production of testosterone and reduce sperm production.
Reduced Sperm Quality: Stress can lead to oxidative damage, causing sperm DNA fragmentation, decreased motility, and lower chances of fertilization.

How to Manage Stress:
Practice Relaxation Techniques: Incorporate mindfulness, meditation, yoga, or deep breathing exercises into your daily routine to reduce stress and lower cortisol levels.
Exercise: Regular physical activity is a powerful way to reduce stress and improve mental well-being.
Sleep Well: Prioritize quality sleep to support hormone regulation and reduce stress levels.

Exposure to Environmental Toxins
Environmental toxins, such as chemicals found in pesticides, plastics, and household cleaning products, can disrupt hormonal balance and negatively affect sperm health. Exposure to

endocrine-disrupting chemicals (EDCs) has been linked to reduced sperm count and quality.

How Toxins Affect Sperm Health:
Hormonal Disruption: Many environmental toxins mimic or interfere with the body's natural hormones, leading to reduced testosterone levels and impaired sperm production.
Sperm DNA Damage: Certain chemicals can cause oxidative stress, leading to DNA fragmentation in sperm cells and reducing fertility.

How to Avoid Exposure to Toxins:
Choose Natural Products: Opt for natural cleaning products, personal care items, and pesticides to reduce exposure to harmful chemicals.
Avoid BPA: BPA (bisphenol A), found in many plastics, is an endocrine disruptor. Use BPA-free products and avoid storing food in plastic containers.
Limit Exposure to Pollutants: Minimize exposure to air pollution and chemicals by choosing organic food and avoiding environmental toxins when possible.

Avoiding harmful habits is key to maintaining optimal sperm health and fertility. By quitting smoking, limiting alcohol intake, avoiding excessive heat exposure, maintaining a healthy diet, staying physically active, managing stress, and reducing exposure to toxins, men can significantly improve their chances of conception. Making small but consistent changes to lifestyle habits can have a lasting impact on reproductive health, supporting healthy sperm count, motility, and overall fertility.

CHAPTER 8

Medical Support and Professional Guidance

When it comes to improving sperm health and fertility, medical support and professional guidance can provide valuable insights and tailored recommendations. While lifestyle changes and natural remedies play a significant role, consulting with a healthcare provider ensures a comprehensive approach to improving reproductive health.

Consulting a Healthcare Provider

If you're concerned about your sperm health or fertility, the first step is to consult with a healthcare provider. A doctor, specifically a urologist or a fertility specialist (andrologist), can help evaluate your reproductive health and provide guidance on improving sperm count and quality. These specialists are trained to diagnose and treat male infertility and can offer personalized recommendations based on your individual health history and lifestyle.

What to Expect During a Consultation:

Medical History Review: Your healthcare provider will start by asking about your medical history, lifestyle habits, family history of fertility issues, and any previous health conditions (such as diabetes, obesity, or testicular injuries) that might impact fertility.

Physical Examination: A physical exam will help the doctor assess your overall health, including any signs of hormonal imbalances, varicocele (enlarged veins in the scrotum), or other conditions that might affect sperm production.

Semen Analysis: One of the most common tests for assessing sperm health is a semen analysis. This test measures sperm count, motility, morphology (shape), and volume of the semen. The results of this test can help determine the cause of infertility and guide the treatment plan.

Blood Tests: Your doctor may recommend blood tests to check hormone levels, such as testosterone, follicle-stimulating hormone (FSH), and luteinizing hormone (LH). These tests help assess whether hormonal imbalances are contributing to low sperm count or quality.

Scrotal Ultrasound: In some cases, a scrotal ultrasound may be performed to check for issues like varicocele or blockages in the reproductive tract that could impair sperm production or delivery.

Fertility Treatments and Interventions

If lifestyle changes alone do not resolve sperm health issues, there are several medical treatments and interventions available. These treatments may be recommended by a fertility specialist based on the underlying cause of sperm health problems.

Medications for Hormonal Imbalances:
Clomiphene Citrate (Clomid): Clomid is a medication often used to treat male infertility caused by hormonal imbalances. It works by stimulating the pituitary gland to increase the production of testosterone and other hormones that support sperm production.
Human Chorionic Gonadotropin (hCG): hCG is sometimes used in combination with other medications to treat men with low testosterone levels or those who have low sperm count due to pituitary issues. It helps stimulate the testes to produce sperm and testosterone.
Gonadotropins: In some cases, gonadotropins (FSH and LH) may be prescribed to stimulate the production of sperm in men who have low sperm count due to a hormonal imbalance or pituitary disorder.

Surgical Interventions:
Varicocele Repair: A varicocele is a condition where the veins in the scrotum become enlarged, leading to reduced sperm production and quality. Surgery to repair varicocele can improve sperm count and quality in some men.
Sperm Retrieval: For men with very low sperm count or no sperm in their semen, procedures like

testicular sperm extraction (TESE) or percutaneous epididymal sperm aspiration (PESA) can be performed. These procedures allow doctors to extract sperm directly from the testes or epididymis for use in assisted reproductive technologies, such as in vitro fertilization (IVF).

Assisted Reproductive Technologies (ART):
In cases where natural conception is not possible due to sperm issues, assisted reproductive technologies (ART) can be used to help achieve pregnancy.

Intrauterine Insemination (IUI): IUI involves placing sperm directly into the uterus during ovulation. This procedure can be used for men with mild sperm issues, such as low sperm count or motility.
In Vitro Fertilization (IVF): IVF is a more advanced ART procedure where sperm is used to fertilize an egg outside the body. IVF is often recommended for men with severe sperm issues, such as very low sperm count or sperm quality.
Intracytoplasmic Sperm Injection (ICSI): ICSI is a specialized form of IVF where a single sperm is injected directly into an egg. This procedure is often used in cases of male infertility when sperm count or motility is very low.

Genetic Counseling and Testing
In some cases, male infertility may have a genetic component. If you have a history of infertility in your

family, or if sperm count and quality issues are unexplained, genetic testing may be recommended. Genetic counseling can help determine if there are hereditary factors contributing to infertility.

Types of Genetic Testing:
Karyotyping: Karyotyping is a test that examines the chromosomes to check for abnormalities. This can help identify conditions like Klinefelter syndrome (an extra X chromosome) or Y chromosome microdeletions, which can lead to infertility.
Y-Chromosome Microdeletion Testing: Y-chromosome microdeletions can lead to low sperm count or infertility. This test examines the Y chromosome for small deletions that may be contributing to sperm production issues.
Cystic Fibrosis Carrier Screening: Men with a history of infertility may be tested for cystic fibrosis mutations, as some men with cystic fibrosis may have no sperm or severely reduced sperm count.

Lifestyle and Wellness Support
In addition to medical treatments, healthcare providers may recommend lifestyle changes to improve sperm health. These may include advice on improving diet, reducing stress, and incorporating regular exercise to enhance fertility.

Diet and Nutrition Guidance:
Consult a Nutritionist: A nutritionist or dietitian can provide tailored dietary recommendations to support

sperm health. This may include increasing intake of antioxidants, vitamins (such as Vitamin C, E, and D), and minerals like zinc, selenium, and folate that are known to improve sperm health.
Weight Management: If overweight or obese, a healthcare provider may recommend a weight loss plan to help improve hormonal balance and sperm production.

Stress Management and Mental Health Support:
Therapy: Chronic stress can have a significant impact on sperm count and quality. A therapist specializing in fertility counseling can help you manage stress and anxiety related to fertility challenges.
Mindfulness and Relaxation Techniques: Techniques like yoga, meditation, or deep breathing exercises can help lower cortisol levels and improve overall reproductive health.

When to Seek Professional Help
It's recommended that men seek medical support if:

You have been trying to conceive for over a year without success (or 6 months if you are over 35 years old).
You have a history of health conditions that might affect fertility (e.g., diabetes, hypertension, or testicular problems).

You have lifestyle factors (such as smoking or excessive alcohol use) that could impact sperm health.
You experience symptoms like erectile dysfunction, pain or swelling in the testicles, or a noticeable decrease in libido.

Medical support and professional guidance are essential for addressing sperm health and fertility concerns. Consulting a healthcare provider, such as a urologist or fertility specialist, allows for a thorough evaluation of sperm count and quality. Depending on the diagnosis, treatments such as medications, surgery, or assisted reproductive technologies may be recommended. Additionally, lifestyle changes, such as improved diet and stress management, play a key role in optimizing sperm health. Working with healthcare professionals ensures that you receive a personalized and comprehensive approach to improving fertility and achieving your reproductive goals.

CHAPTER 9

The Journey to Fertility

Fertility is a complex and personal journey, and when faced with challenges, it can often feel overwhelming. However, understanding the process, being proactive about health, and seeking the right support can help guide the way toward successful conception.

Understanding Fertility: A Holistic Approach

Fertility is influenced by a combination of physical, hormonal, and lifestyle factors. For men, sperm count, motility (ability to move), morphology (shape), and overall health are the key indicators of fertility. In addition to sperm health, overall wellness, stress levels, and external factors such as environmental toxins also play a crucial role.

Fertility is not just a single factor but a combination of elements that work together to achieve conception. This holistic view involves addressing all aspects of health—nutrition, exercise, mental well-being, and medical care—to create the best environment for sperm production and successful fertilization.

The Initial Steps: Evaluation and Assessment
The journey to fertility often begins with a comprehensive evaluation. For men facing challenges in conceiving, a medical check-up is essential to identify any potential issues that may be contributing to low sperm count or fertility problems. A visit to a fertility specialist, urologist, or andrologist will typically include the following steps:

a. Medical History and Physical Examination
Your healthcare provider will ask about your medical history, lifestyle, and any potential environmental or genetic factors that could affect fertility. This includes discussing:

Previous health conditions (e.g., diabetes, high blood pressure, or past surgeries).
Family history of infertility.
Lifestyle habits like smoking, alcohol consumption, and exercise.
Symptoms like erectile dysfunction or pain in the testicles.
A physical exam will assess signs of hormonal imbalances, varicocele (enlarged veins in the scrotum), and any other issues that may impact sperm health.

b. Semen Analysis
The semen analysis is the cornerstone of fertility testing for men. It evaluates several key factors of sperm health:

Sperm Count: The number of sperm in the sample.
Motility: The percentage of sperm that are actively moving.
Morphology: The shape of the sperm, as abnormally shaped sperm can affect their ability to fertilize an egg.
Volume and pH: These tests measure the amount and the acidity of the semen.
This test will give the doctor a clear picture of sperm health and determine if further investigation or treatment is needed.

c. Hormonal and Blood Tests
Blood tests can evaluate hormone levels, such as testosterone, follicle-stimulating hormone (FSH), and luteinizing hormone (LH). Hormonal imbalances, such as low testosterone or high prolactin levels, can affect sperm production and require treatment.

Optimizing Sperm Health: Lifestyle Adjustments
Once the medical assessment is complete, it's time to take proactive steps to improve sperm health. While medical treatments are available for specific conditions, lifestyle changes can significantly enhance fertility and contribute to better sperm quality and overall reproductive health.

a. Nutrition and Diet
The foods you eat play a crucial role in sperm health. A balanced diet rich in antioxidants, vitamins,

and minerals can help protect sperm from oxidative stress and support healthy sperm production. Focus on:

Antioxidant-Rich Foods: Berries, nuts, seeds, and leafy greens are rich in antioxidants, which protect sperm from free radical damage.
Healthy Fats: Omega-3 fatty acids, found in fish, flaxseeds, and walnuts, are known to support sperm motility.
Essential Vitamins and Minerals: Zinc, selenium, vitamin C, vitamin D, and folate are essential for sperm health. Foods like eggs, shellfish, citrus fruits, and fortified cereals can provide these nutrients.
Limit Processed Foods: Avoid high sugar, high-fat, and processed foods, which can lead to inflammation and hormonal imbalances.

b. Physical Activity
Regular exercise not only supports overall health but also improves blood circulation, hormone regulation, and stress management. Moderate physical activity, such as walking, swimming, or cycling, can enhance sperm quality.

However, it's important to find a balance. Excessive exercise, especially intense activities like long-distance running or heavy weightlifting, can lead to hormonal imbalances and reduced sperm production.

c. Weight Management
Being overweight or obese can disrupt hormone levels and reduce sperm count and motility. Losing excess weight through a healthy diet and exercise can improve fertility outcomes. Aim for a body mass index (BMI) within the healthy range to support optimal sperm production.

d. Stress Reduction
Chronic stress can elevate cortisol levels, which negatively affects sperm production and motility. Implementing stress reduction techniques, such as mindfulness, meditation, yoga, or deep breathing exercises, can help lower stress hormones and improve overall reproductive health.

e. Adequate Sleep and Hydration
Getting 7–9 hours of quality sleep per night is essential for maintaining hormonal balance and overall health. Poor sleep is linked to lower testosterone levels and decreased sperm count.

Staying hydrated is equally important. Dehydration can lead to a decrease in semen volume and quality, so aim to drink plenty of water throughout the day.

Seeking Medical Support: When to Take the Next Step
While lifestyle changes are essential, they may not always be sufficient, especially if there are underlying medical conditions affecting sperm

production. In such cases, it's important to seek professional medical treatment. Depending on the results of semen analysis and other tests, a healthcare provider may recommend the following:

a. Medications
Clomiphene Citrate: This medication can help boost testosterone production in men with low testosterone levels, increasing sperm count.
Gonadotropins: If low levels of FSH or LH are causing low sperm production, gonadotropin injections may stimulate sperm production.
Antioxidants: Some doctors may prescribe antioxidant supplements to reduce oxidative stress and improve sperm health.

b. Surgery
Varicocele Repair: If you have a varicocele (swollen veins in the scrotum), surgical correction may improve sperm production and motility.
Sperm Retrieval: If sperm count is extremely low or absent, sperm may be retrieved surgically through methods like TESE (testicular sperm extraction) or PESA (percutaneous epididymal sperm aspiration).

c. Assisted Reproductive Technologies (ART)
For couples who are unable to conceive naturally, ART options like Intrauterine Insemination (IUI), In Vitro Fertilization (IVF), and Intracytoplasmic Sperm Injection (ICSI) are available. These methods can increase the chances of successful fertilization by

directly addressing sperm count, motility, or egg fertilization issues.

Emotional Support and Mental Well-Being
The journey to fertility can be emotionally challenging. The pressure of trying to conceive, combined with potential setbacks, can lead to feelings of frustration, anxiety, or depression. It's important to prioritize mental well-being during this time.

Couples Counseling: Fertility issues can place a strain on relationships. Counseling or fertility therapy can help couples manage emotional stress and strengthen their bond.
Support Groups: Connecting with others who are going through similar experiences can provide a sense of community and support.
Mindfulness and Relaxation: Practicing mindfulness, yoga, and meditation can reduce anxiety and improve overall well-being.

Maintaining Hope and Patience
Fertility journeys often take time, and it's important to be patient with the process. Even with the best medical care and lifestyle improvements, it may take several months or longer to see results. Maintaining hope and focusing on the small steps along the way can help you stay motivated and optimistic about achieving your fertility goals.

Conclusion: The Path to Fertility Is Personal
The journey to fertility is unique for each individual and couple. It involves a combination of lifestyle changes, medical support, emotional well-being, and, in some cases, assisted reproductive technologies. By taking a holistic approach—focusing on optimizing sperm health through diet, exercise, stress reduction, and medical treatment—you can improve your chances of conception and navigate this challenging yet rewarding path to parenthood.

CHAPTER 10

Conclusion

Achieving and maintaining a healthy sperm count naturally is a process that involves a multi-faceted approach, combining lifestyle adjustments, nutrition, stress management, and, when necessary, medical interventions. By focusing on overall health and making informed choices, it's possible to enhance fertility, improve sperm quality, and increase the chances of successful conception.

Long-Term Maintenance for Optimal Fertility

Sperm health is not a one-time fix but a long-term commitment to maintaining a healthy lifestyle and staying proactive about your reproductive health. Even after achieving a healthy sperm count, it's essential to continue the habits that support fertility. This includes:

Consistent Healthy Eating: Continue to consume a balanced diet rich in antioxidants, vitamins, minerals, and healthy fats that support sperm production.
Regular Exercise: Moderate physical activity helps maintain healthy blood flow, hormone levels, and weight, which are key to sustaining sperm health.
Stress Management: Continue using stress-reduction techniques like meditation, yoga, and

therapy to manage anxiety and cortisol levels, which can impact sperm production.

Adequate Sleep: Consistently get 7–9 hours of quality sleep to maintain hormonal balance and overall well-being.

Avoid Harmful Toxins: Limit exposure to environmental toxins such as chemicals, pesticides, and pollutants that can damage sperm cells and impair fertility.

Routine Health Check-ups: Regular visits to your healthcare provider, especially if you have underlying health conditions, can ensure that any fertility issues are caught early.

By making these practices a consistent part of your daily routine, you can maintain a high level of sperm health and improve your overall fertility.

Final Thoughts and Next Steps

Achieving a healthy sperm count and optimal fertility is a journey that requires time, patience, and dedication. It's important to remember that everyone's fertility journey is unique, and what works for one person may not be the solution for another. The key is to stay informed, be proactive, and seek the appropriate medical support when necessary.

If you are experiencing fertility challenges, remember that you are not alone. Consult with a healthcare provider to get a personalized treatment plan based on your individual needs. Whether it involves lifestyle changes, medical treatments, or assisted reproductive technologies, there are various paths to achieving your fertility goals.

Next Steps:
Begin with a Consultation: If you haven't already, schedule a consultation with a fertility specialist to assess your sperm health and discuss potential options for treatment.

Implement Healthy Habits: Start incorporating changes in diet, exercise, and stress management to create an optimal environment for sperm production.

Monitor Progress: Stay consistent with your fertility-boosting practices and monitor any changes in your health and sperm quality over time.

Stay Hopeful and Patient: Fertility journeys can take time. Stay hopeful and patient as you navigate your path toward achieving a healthy sperm count and conception.

Your fertility journey is an ongoing process of discovery, adaptation, and growth. By staying dedicated to improving your health and seeking the right support, you can optimize your chances of achieving your reproductive goals. Keep moving forward, and remember that each step you take brings you closer to your desired outcome.